Kloe Steele

The Power of Nature: Essential Oils, Herbs, and Homeopathy for Stress and Anxiety Relief

Table Of Contents

Building a Homeopathic First Aid Kit

Chapter 1: Understanding Stress and Anxiety

The Impact of Stress and Anxiety on Health

In today's fast-paced world, stress and anxiety have become all too common. The pressures of modern life can take a toll on our mental and physical well-being, affecting every aspect of our lives. In this subchapter, we will explore the profound impact that stress and anxiety can have on our health and how utilizing essential oils and herbs can provide relief.

Stress and anxiety have been linked to a wide range of health problems, from cardiovascular issues to immune system disorders. When we are constantly in a state of stress, our bodies produce an excess of cortisol, the stress hormone. This can lead to high blood pressure, increased heart rate, and even heart disease. Moreover, chronic stress weakens our immune system, making us more susceptible to illnesses and infections.

The effects of stress and anxiety are not limited to our physical health; they also impact our mental well-being. Prolonged stress can lead to feelings of overwhelm, burnout, and depression. It can hinder our ability to concentrate, affect our memory, and disrupt sleep patterns. In essence, stress and anxiety can diminish our overall quality of life.

Fortunately, there are natural remedies available to help combat stress and anxiety. Essential oils, such as lavender, chamomile, and bergamot, have been used for centuries to promote relaxation and ease emotional distress. These oils can be diffused, applied topically, or added to bathwater to create a soothing and calming atmosphere.

Similarly, certain herbs have been found to have stress-reducing properties. Adaptogenic herbs like ashwagandha and holy basil help the body adapt to stress and restore balance. They can be consumed as supplements or brewed into teas for a holistic approach to stress relief.

Homeopathy, a system of medicine based on the principle of "like cures like," offers a unique approach to managing stress and anxiety. Homeopathic remedies, derived from natural substances, are tailored to the individual's specific symptoms and emotions. These remedies can help restore harmony within the body and alleviate the effects of stress and anxiety.

By incorporating essential oils, herbs, and homeopathy into your self-care routine, you can effectively address the impact of stress and anxiety on your health. The power of nature provides us with gentle yet potent tools to promote relaxation, restore balance, and enhance our overall well-being. Embracing these natural remedies allows us to take control of our health and find relief from the pressures of modern life.

The Mind-Body Connection

In today's fast-paced world, stress and anxiety have become increasingly common. Many individuals are seeking natural remedies to alleviate these burdens and restore a sense of calm and balance to their lives. One powerful approach that has gained significant attention is the mind-body connection, which recognizes the profound influence our thoughts and emotions have on our physical well-being. In this subchapter, we will explore how to harness the power of nature, specifically essential oils, herbs, and homeopathy, to address stress and anxiety through the mind-body connection.

The Power of Nature: Essential Oils, Herbs, and Homeopathy for Stress and Anxiety Relief

Understanding the mind-body connection is essential to effectively managing stress and anxiety. Research has shown that our thoughts and emotions can directly impact our physical health, leading to imbalances and ailments. By acknowledging this connection, we can begin to utilize the healing properties of essential oils, herbs, and homeopathy to restore harmony within ourselves.

Essential oils, derived from plants and their aromatic compounds, have been used for centuries to promote relaxation, relieve tension, and uplift the spirit. Lavender, for example, is renowned for its calming properties and can be diffused or applied topically to reduce stress and anxiety. Similarly, chamomile and bergamot oils have proven to be effective in soothing the mind and promoting emotional well-being. By incorporating these oils into our daily self-care routines, we can tap into their therapeutic benefits and support our mental and physical health.

Herbs, too, hold immense potential in combating stress and anxiety. Adaptogenic herbs such as ashwagandha and holy basil have long been used in traditional medicine to help the body adapt to stressors and promote relaxation. Additionally, herbs like lemon balm, passionflower, and valerian root can aid in calming the nervous system and improving sleep quality. By incorporating these herbs into teas, tinctures, or capsules, individuals can experience their natural healing properties and find relief from the burdens of stress and anxiety.

Homeopathy, a system of medicine based on the principle of "like cures like," offers unique remedies for stress and anxiety relief. Homeopathic remedies are derived from natural substances and work to stimulate the body's innate healing abilities. These remedies can help address the underlying causes of stress and anxiety, such as fear, restlessness, or overwhelming emotions. By consulting with a qualified homeopath, individuals can discover personalized remedies that resonate with their specific symptoms and experiences.

In conclusion, the mind-body connection is a powerful tool in the realm of stress and anxiety relief. By utilizing essential oils, herbs, and homeopathy, individuals can tap into the healing potential of nature and restore balance to their lives. Whether through diffusing calming scents, sipping herbal teas, or exploring personalized homeopathic remedies, individuals interested in self-care with homeopathy can find solace in the power of nature. Embracing the mind-body connection is a transformative journey towards cultivating inner peace and well-being.

Identifying Symptoms and Triggers

In the fast-paced world we live in, stress and anxiety have become all too common. Many individuals are seeking natural remedies to alleviate these overwhelming feelings and regain control of their lives. Essential oils, herbs, and homeopathy offer a holistic approach to stress and anxiety relief, allowing individuals to find peace and balance amidst the chaos.

But before diving into the world of natural remedies, it is crucial to understand and identify the symptoms and triggers that contribute to your stress and anxiety. By recognizing these signs, you can tailor your self-care routine with essential oils and herbs to target specific areas and achieve optimal results.

The Power of Nature: Essential Oils, Herbs, and Homeopathy for Stress and Anxiety Relief

Symptoms of stress and anxiety can manifest both physically and mentally. On a physical level, you may experience tension headaches, muscle aches, fatigue, or even digestive issues. Mentally, you might find yourself constantly worrying, feeling overwhelmed, or having trouble concentrating. By paying attention to these indicators, you can gain valuable insight into your body's response to stress, allowing you to take proactive steps towards relieving them.

Triggers are the underlying causes behind your stress and anxiety. They can vary greatly from person to person, but some common triggers include work-related pressure, financial concerns, relationship issues, or even traumatic experiences. Identifying these triggers is essential as it enables you to address the root causes of your stress and anxiety, rather than merely treating the symptoms.

Once you have identified your symptoms and triggers, you can explore the world of essential oils and herbs to find the perfect remedies for your unique needs. Lavender, for example, is renowned for its calming properties and can be used to alleviate anxiety and promote a peaceful sleep. Chamomile tea, on the other hand, is a gentle herb that can soothe your nerves and induce relaxation.

Homeopathy, a natural system of medicine, offers a wide range of remedies tailored to individual symptoms and triggers. By consulting with a homeopath, you can discover personalized solutions that address both the physical and emotional aspects of your stress and anxiety.

In this subchapter, we will explore various symptoms and triggers associated with stress and anxiety. We will delve into the powerful effects of essential oils, herbs, and homeopathy in alleviating these conditions. By gaining a deeper understanding of your own stress and anxiety, you can embark on a journey of self-care and empowerment, utilizing the incredible power of nature to find relief and achieve a balanced, fulfilling life.

Chapter 2: Introduction to Essential Oils

What are Essential Oils?

Essential oils are highly concentrated plant extracts that capture the aromatic properties and beneficial compounds of various plants. They have been used for centuries in traditional medicine practices and are renowned for their therapeutic properties. In the realm of self-care, essential oils offer a natural and holistic approach to alleviating stress and anxiety, making them a valuable tool for individuals seeking alternative methods for relaxation and well-being.

Derived from different parts of plants including flowers, leaves, stems, and roots, essential oils are obtained through a process of steam distillation or cold pressing. This extraction method ensures that the final product contains the purest and most potent essence of the plant. The resulting oil retains the characteristic fragrance and therapeutic properties of the plant it originates from, allowing users to experience the benefits of nature in a concentrated form.

The Power of Nature: Essential Oils, Herbs, and Homeopathy for Stress and Anxiety Relief

One of the most fascinating aspects of essential oils is their ability to affect our emotions and mood. When inhaled or applied to the skin, essential oils can help calm the mind, uplift the spirit, and promote a sense of relaxation. They work by interacting with the limbic system, the part of our brain responsible for emotions and memory. This makes essential oils a powerful tool in managing stress and anxiety.

There are a wide variety of essential oils available, each with its own unique properties and benefits. Lavender, for example, is known for its calming and balancing effects, while citrus oils like lemon and orange can invigorate and uplift the senses. Eucalyptus and peppermint are often used for their refreshing and clearing properties, especially when dealing with respiratory issues caused by stress.

To utilize essential oils effectively, it is essential to understand their various applications. They can be used in aromatherapy, where the oils are diffused into the air or inhaled directly from the bottle. They can also be applied topically, either in diluted form or blended with carrier oils, to target specific areas of the body.

In this book, "The Power of Nature: Essential Oils, Herbs, and Homeopathy for Stress and Anxiety Relief," we will explore the world of essential oils and delve into their potential to support self-care and promote well-being. Whether you are new to essential oils or an experienced user, this book will provide you with valuable insights, practical tips, and evidence-based information to help you harness the power of nature in managing stress and anxiety. So, let's embark on this journey together and discover the transformative potential of essential oils in our lives.

How Essential Oils Work

The Power of Nature: Essential Oils, Herbs, and Homeopathy for Stress and Anxiety Relief

Understanding how essential oils work is essential for anyone interested in self-care with homeopathy. These natural extracts from plants have been used for centuries to promote physical and emotional well-being. In this subchapter, we will explore the mechanisms behind the effectiveness of essential oils in relieving stress and anxiety.

Essential oils are highly concentrated plant extracts derived from various parts of plants, such as flowers, leaves, bark, and roots. They contain volatile compounds that give them their characteristic aroma and therapeutic properties. When inhaled or applied topically, these compounds interact with our bodies in several ways.

One of the primary modes of action of essential oils is through the olfactory system. When we inhale the aroma of essential oils, the molecules travel through the nose and reach the olfactory receptors. These receptors send signals to the limbic system, the part of the brain responsible for emotions and memories. This direct connection to the limbic system explains why essential oils can have such a profound impact on our mood and emotions.

Furthermore, essential oils can also be absorbed through the skin when applied topically. The skin acts as a barrier, but certain essential oil molecules are small enough to penetrate and enter the bloodstream. Once in the bloodstream, they can exert their therapeutic effects throughout the body. For example, lavender essential oil has been shown to reduce anxiety by modulating the activity of neurotransmitters such as serotonin and GABA.

Additionally, essential oils possess antimicrobial, anti-inflammatory, and antioxidant properties. These properties can support the body's natural healing processes and help reduce stress-related symptoms. For instance, studies have demonstrated the anxiolytic effects of chamomile essential oil, which can help promote relaxation and improve sleep quality.

It's important to note that while essential oils can be beneficial for stress and anxiety relief, they are not a substitute for professional medical advice. They should be used as part of a holistic approach to self-care, which may include other practices such as meditation, exercise, and a balanced diet.

By understanding how essential oils work, individuals interested in self-care with homeopathy can harness the power of nature to support their well-being. Incorporating essential oils into daily routines, such as diffusing them in the home or using them in massages, can provide a natural and effective way to reduce stress and anxiety, promoting a sense of calm and balance in one's life.

Safety Precautions and Guidelines

When it comes to utilizing essential oils, herbs, and homeopathy for stress and anxiety relief, it is crucial to prioritize safety and adhere to certain guidelines. While these natural remedies can be highly effective, it is essential to use them responsibly and with caution. This subchapter will provide you with important safety precautions and guidelines to ensure a safe and enjoyable self-care experience.

1. Dilution: Essential oils are highly concentrated substances and should never be applied directly to the skin without dilution. Always dilute essential oils with a carrier oil, such as coconut or jojoba oil, before applying topically. This helps to prevent skin irritation and sensitization.

2. Patch Test: Before applying any essential oil or herbal remedy to a larger area on your body, it is advisable to perform a patch test. Apply a small amount of the diluted mixture to a small area of your skin and observe for any adverse reactions like redness, itching, or irritation. If any negative reactions occur, do not continue using the product.

3. Quality Matters: Ensure that you are using high-quality, pure essential oils and herbs from reputable sources. Look for products that are organic, non-GMO, and have undergone third-party testing to ensure their purity and potency. This will ensure the best results and minimize the risk of adverse effects.

4. Dosage: Always follow the recommended dosage guidelines provided by professionals or reputable sources. It is important to remember that more is not always better when it comes to natural remedies. Using excessive amounts of essential oils or herbs can lead to adverse effects and may not provide better results.

5. Pregnancy and Children: Pregnant women and children require special considerations when using essential oils and herbs. Some oils and herbs may not be safe for use during pregnancy or on young children. It is best to consult with a qualified healthcare professional or a certified aromatherapist to determine which remedies are safe and appropriate for these specific populations.

6. Storage: Proper storage of essential oils and herbs is crucial to maintain their potency and prevent degradation. Store them in dark, glass containers in a cool, dry place away from direct sunlight. This helps to extend their shelf life and ensures that they remain effective.

By following these safety precautions and guidelines, you can confidently incorporate essential oils, herbs, and homeopathy into your self-care routine. Remember, it is always advisable to consult with a healthcare professional or an experienced practitioner if you have any concerns or questions regarding the use of these natural remedies.

Chapter 3: Popular Essential Oils for Stress and Anxiety Relief

Lavender: The Calming Oil

In the bustling world we live in today, it's no surprise that stress and anxiety have become increasingly common issues. From demanding work schedules to personal responsibilities, our minds and bodies are constantly on high alert. But what if there was a natural solution to help us find a sense of calm and relaxation? Enter lavender essential oil, also known as the "calming oil."

Lavender has been used for centuries for its soothing properties. Its gentle scent has the power to transport us to a place of tranquility, easing our worries and helping us unwind. This versatile oil can be a game-changer in your self-care routine, providing relief from stress and anxiety in a safe and natural way.

One of the most effective ways to utilize lavender is through aromatherapy. Simply adding a few drops of lavender essential oil to a diffuser or inhaling it directly from the bottle can work wonders for your mental well-being. The aroma of lavender has been shown to promote relaxation, reduce nervous tension, and even improve sleep quality. It's like having a spa day in the comfort of your own home!

But lavender's benefits don't stop at aromatherapy. This incredible oil can also be used topically to soothe the body and mind. Diluting a few drops of lavender essential oil with a carrier oil, such as coconut or jojoba oil, can create a calming massage blend. Gently massaging this mixture onto your temples, neck, or wrists can help alleviate tension and promote a sense of calmness throughout your body.

Additionally, lavender can be incorporated into your daily skincare routine. Its anti-inflammatory and antibacterial properties make it an excellent choice for soothing irritated skin or treating acne. By adding a few drops of lavender essential oil to your favorite face cleanser or moisturizer, you can enjoy both the physical and mental benefits of this amazing oil.

When it comes to stress and anxiety relief, lavender essential oil is a true powerhouse. Its calming properties can help alleviate feelings of tension, promote relaxation, and create an overall sense of well-being. By incorporating lavender into your self-care routine, you can harness the power of nature to find balance and harmony in your life.

So, go ahead and embrace the calming benefits of lavender. Let its gentle scent transport you to a place of serenity and allow it to guide you on your journey towards stress and anxiety relief. Your mind and body will thank you for it.

Chamomile: Soothing Nerves and Promoting Relaxation

Chamomile, with its delicate white flowers and gentle fragrance, has been used for centuries to calm the mind and relax the body. This remarkable herb is a true powerhouse when it comes to soothing nerves and promoting relaxation, making it an essential addition to your self-care routine.

The Power of Nature: Essential Oils, Herbs, and Homeopathy for Stress and Anxiety Relief

Known for its calming properties, chamomile has long been used as a natural remedy for stress and anxiety relief. Whether you're feeling overwhelmed by the pressures of daily life or struggling to find restful sleep, chamomile can be a valuable ally in restoring balance and tranquility.

One of the most popular ways to utilize chamomile is through its essential oil. By diffusing chamomile oil in your home or office, you can create a peaceful and serene atmosphere that helps to alleviate stress and anxiety. The soothing aroma of chamomile oil can also help to combat insomnia, allowing you to enjoy a restful night's sleep.

Chamomile tea is another wonderful way to harness the calming properties of this herb. By steeping chamomile flowers in hot water, you can create a soothing beverage that promotes relaxation and eases tension. Sipping on a cup of chamomile tea before bed can be particularly beneficial for those struggling with insomnia or restless nights.

In addition to its calming effects, chamomile also possesses anti-inflammatory properties that can help to reduce muscle tension and ease physical discomfort. Whether you're dealing with headaches, menstrual cramps, or general body aches, chamomile can provide much-needed relief.

When it comes to self-care with homeopathy, chamomile is a must-have herb in your arsenal. Its ability to soothe nerves, promote relaxation, and alleviate stress is truly remarkable. Whether you choose to incorporate chamomile essential oil into your daily routine or enjoy a cup of chamomile tea before bed, this herb has the power to transform your well-being.

Remember, self-care is not a luxury but a necessity. By embracing the power of nature and utilizing essential oils and herbs like chamomile, you can take control of your stress and anxiety levels, promoting a healthier and more balanced life.

So why wait? Start incorporating chamomile into your self-care routine today and experience the soothing benefits it has to offer. Your mind, body, and spirit will thank you.

Bergamot: Uplifting and Balancing Emotions

In the quest for stress and anxiety relief, the power of nature offers a wide array of remedies, including essential oils, herbs, and homeopathy. One such remarkable essential oil is bergamot, known for its ability to uplift and balance emotions. This subchapter explores the benefits and applications of bergamot for individuals interested in self-care with homeopathy.

Bergamot, derived from the Citrus bergamia tree, is a small citrus fruit that resembles a cross between a lemon and an orange. Its refreshing and uplifting aroma has been used for centuries to promote emotional well-being. The key component responsible for bergamot's therapeutic properties is its high content of a unique compound called linalool. Linalool is known to possess calming and mood-enhancing effects, making bergamot an ideal choice for stress and anxiety relief.

One of the most effective ways to harness the benefits of bergamot is through aromatherapy. Adding a few drops of bergamot essential oil to a diffuser or inhaling it directly from the bottle can quickly uplift your mood and create a sense of tranquility. The soothing fragrance of bergamot can help alleviate symptoms of anxiety, depression, and even insomnia.

Bergamot can also be used topically, although it is essential to dilute it with a carrier oil such as coconut or jojoba oil to avoid skin irritation. Massaging a diluted mixture onto your temples, wrists, or the back of your neck can provide immediate relief from stress and tension. Additionally, bergamot is known to have antibacterial properties, making it an excellent choice for promoting healthy skin.

For those interested in homeopathy, bergamot can be taken orally in the form of a tincture or as part of a custom-made homeopathic remedy. It is believed to balance the emotions, reduce nervousness, and promote a sense of calmness from within.

However, it is important to note that bergamot essential oil can increase photosensitivity, making your skin more prone to sunburn. Therefore, it is advisable to avoid direct sunlight or use sunscreen after applying bergamot topically.

In conclusion, bergamot is a valuable tool in the realm of stress and anxiety relief. Its uplifting and balancing effects on emotions make it an excellent choice for individuals interested in self-care with homeopathy. Whether through aromatherapy, topical application, or homeopathic remedies, bergamot can bring harmony and tranquility to your daily life. Embrace the power of nature and let bergamot be your ally in finding emotional well-being.

Ylang Ylang: Easing Tension and Promoting Tranquility

In the pursuit of self-care and relief from stress and anxiety, essential oils and herbs have emerged as powerful allies. One such gem is ylang ylang, a fragrant flower known for its ability to ease tension and promote tranquility. In this subchapter, we will delve into the wonders of ylang ylang and explore its countless benefits in the realm of homeopathy.

The Power of Nature: Essential Oils, Herbs, and Homeopathy for Stress and Anxiety Relief

Originating from the lush forests of Southeast Asia, ylang ylang possesses a unique aroma that instantly transports you to a state of peace and calm. Its delicate floral scent has long been used in aromatherapy to reduce stress, anxiety, and even symptoms of depression. By simply inhaling its sweet fragrance, you can experience a profound sense of relaxation and emotional balance.

Ylang ylang essential oil, derived from the flowers through a meticulous distillation process, is a versatile remedy for various ailments. Its sedative properties make it an excellent choice for those struggling with insomnia or restless sleep. Just a few drops on your pillow or in a diffuser before bedtime can work wonders in promoting a deep and restful slumber.

In addition to its calming effects on the mind, ylang ylang is also beneficial for physical well-being. It possesses antispasmodic properties that can ease muscle tension and menstrual cramps. By diluting it with a carrier oil and massaging it onto the affected areas, you can experience relief and a sense of comfort.

Furthermore, ylang ylang is believed to have aphrodisiac qualities, enhancing sensuality and intimacy. Its ability to reduce stress and promote relaxation can create an ideal setting for deeper connections and emotional intimacy.

When incorporating ylang ylang into your self-care routine, it is important to remember that essential oils are potent and should be used with caution. Always dilute them properly and perform a patch test before applying them to your skin. If you are pregnant, nursing, or have any underlying medical conditions, it is advisable to consult with a qualified healthcare professional before using ylang ylang or any other essential oils.

In conclusion, ylang ylang is a valuable tool in the journey towards stress and anxiety relief. Its ability to ease tension, promote tranquility, and enhance overall well-being makes it a must-have in your essential oil collection. By harnessing the power of nature through ylang ylang, you can create a sanctuary of calm and find solace in the midst of life's challenges.

Frankincense: Calming the Mind and Enhancing Spiritual Connection

Frankincense has a long and revered history as a powerful tool for calming the mind and enhancing spiritual connection. Derived from the resin of the Boswellia tree, this essential oil has been used for centuries in various cultures for its healing properties. In this subchapter, we will explore the benefits of frankincense in relieving stress and anxiety, and how it can be incorporated into your self-care routine with homeopathy.

One of the key benefits of frankincense is its ability to calm the mind and promote relaxation. Its rich and earthy aroma has a grounding effect, helping to reduce feelings of anxiety and tension. By inhaling the scent of frankincense, you can create a sense of peace and tranquility, allowing your mind to unwind from the stresses of daily life.

In addition to its calming properties, frankincense is also known for its ability to enhance spiritual connection. It has been used in religious and spiritual rituals for centuries, as it is believed to heighten intuition and deepen meditation. By incorporating frankincense into your daily practice, you can create a sacred space for self-reflection and inner exploration.

There are several ways to utilize frankincense for stress and anxiety relief. One popular method is through aromatherapy. You can add a few drops of frankincense essential oil to a diffuser and let the scent fill the room. Alternatively, you can create a calming blend by combining frankincense with other essential oils such as lavender or chamomile.

Another way to incorporate frankincense into your self-care routine is through topical application. Dilute a few drops of frankincense essential oil with a carrier oil, such as coconut or jojoba oil, and massage it onto your temples, wrists, or the soles of your feet. This can help promote relaxation and alleviate feelings of stress.

Lastly, frankincense can also be used in homeopathic remedies for stress and anxiety. Consult with a qualified homeopath to determine the best way to incorporate frankincense into your personalized treatment plan.

In conclusion, frankincense is a powerful tool for calming the mind and enhancing spiritual connection. Whether you choose to use it through aromatherapy, topical application, or homeopathy, incorporating frankincense into your self-care routine can provide immense relief from stress and anxiety. Take the time to explore the benefits of this ancient essential oil and discover the transformative power of nature.

Chapter 4: Utilizing Herbs for Stress and Anxiety Relief

The Benefits of Herbal Remedies

The Power of Nature: Essential Oils, Herbs, and Homeopathy for Stress and Anxiety Relief

In today's fast-paced and stressful world, finding effective ways to manage stress and anxiety is crucial for maintaining overall well-being. While there are many options available, one approach that has gained significant popularity is the use of herbal remedies. This subchapter explores the various benefits of herbal remedies and how they can be utilized for stress and anxiety relief.

Herbal remedies are derived from plants and have been used for centuries in traditional medicine practices. The power of nature is harnessed through essential oils, herbs, and homeopathy, offering a natural and holistic alternative to conventional treatments. For individuals interested in self-care with homeopathy, incorporating herbal remedies into their routine can be a game-changer.

One of the key benefits of herbal remedies is their ability to promote relaxation and reduce stress. Certain herbs, such as lavender and chamomile, are known for their calming properties. These herbs can be used in various forms, including essential oils, teas, or even as supplements, to help individuals unwind and find inner peace amidst the chaos of daily life.

Additionally, herbal remedies can also help alleviate anxiety symptoms. Herbs like valerian root and passionflower have been shown to have anxiolytic effects, reducing feelings of unease and restlessness. By incorporating these herbs into their self-care routine, individuals can experience a natural approach to managing their anxiety without relying solely on pharmaceutical options.

The Power of Nature: Essential Oils, Herbs, and Homeopathy for Stress and Anxiety Relief

Furthermore, herbal remedies offer a gentler and safer alternative to harsh chemical-based medications. Many pharmaceutical drugs for stress and anxiety come with a plethora of side effects, which can be quite debilitating. Herbal remedies, on the other hand, generally have fewer side effects and are considered to be more gentle on the body. This makes them an attractive option for individuals who prefer a more natural and holistic approach to their health.

Finally, herbal remedies can also provide additional benefits beyond stress and anxiety relief. Many herbs possess antioxidant properties, which can help boost the immune system and improve overall well-being. They can also aid in promoting better sleep, enhancing cognitive function, and supporting a healthy digestive system.

In conclusion, the use of herbal remedies offers numerous benefits for individuals interested in self-care with homeopathy. From promoting relaxation and reducing stress to alleviating anxiety symptoms, herbal remedies provide a natural and holistic approach to managing stress and anxiety. With fewer side effects and additional health benefits, incorporating herbal remedies into one's routine can be a powerful tool for achieving overall well-being and finding inner peace in a hectic world.

Preparing Herbal Infusions and Teas

Herbal infusions and teas are excellent natural remedies to help alleviate stress and anxiety. These plant-based remedies have been used for centuries and are known for their calming and soothing properties. In this subchapter, we will explore the art of preparing herbal infusions and teas to harness the power of nature in promoting relaxation and well-being.

To begin, it is essential to understand the difference between herbal infusions and teas. Herbal infusions are made by steeping medicinal herbs in hot water for a longer period, typically 10-20 minutes. Teas, on the other hand, are made by steeping tea leaves or herbs in hot water for a shorter time, usually 3-5 minutes. Both methods extract the beneficial compounds from the herbs, allowing you to enjoy their therapeutic benefits.

When preparing herbal infusions and teas, it is crucial to select high-quality herbs. Look for organic or wildcrafted herbs to ensure their purity and potency. You can find a variety of herbs that are beneficial for stress and anxiety relief, such as chamomile, lavender, lemon balm, passionflower, and holy basil. Each herb has its unique properties, so feel free to experiment and find the ones that resonate with you.

To prepare an herbal infusion, bring water to a boil and pour it over the herbs in a heat-resistant container. Cover the container and let it steep for the recommended time. Once steeped, strain the infusion and enjoy it warm or chilled. You can sweeten it with honey or add a slice of lemon for extra flavor.

For a quick and easy tea, place a tea bag or loose herbs in a cup and pour hot water over them. Let it steep for a few minutes and remove the tea bag or strain the herbs. You can add a touch of honey or a squeeze of lemon to enhance the taste.

Remember, herbal infusions and teas are not only delicious but also powerful allies in your self-care routine. Take the time to sit down, savor your tea, and embrace the calming effects it provides. Incorporating these natural remedies into your daily routine can help you find balance, reduce stress, and alleviate anxiety.

The Power of Nature: Essential Oils, Herbs, and Homeopathy for Stress and Anxiety Relief

In conclusion, preparing herbal infusions and teas is a simple and effective way to tap into the power of nature for stress and anxiety relief. By selecting high-quality herbs and following the proper steeping techniques, you can create delightful and therapeutic beverages to support your well-being. Embrace the tranquility and relaxation that these herbal remedies offer as you embark on your journey of self-care with homeopathy.

Herbs for Relaxation and Calming the Nervous System

In today's fast-paced world, stress and anxiety have become a common part of our daily lives. As individuals interested in self-care with homeopathy, it is essential to explore natural remedies that can help us find relaxation and restore balance to our nervous system. This subchapter focuses on the power of herbs in achieving this goal.

Herbs have been used for centuries to promote relaxation and calmness. They offer a gentle and effective alternative to pharmaceuticals, with minimal side effects. By incorporating these herbs into our daily routine, we can create a nurturing and soothing environment for our mind and body.

One of the most popular herbs for relaxation is chamomile. Known for its gentle sedative effects, chamomile tea is a wonderful way to unwind after a long day. Its calming properties can help reduce anxiety and promote better sleep. Similarly, lavender, with its delightful aroma, has been used for centuries to induce relaxation and relieve stress. Whether in the form of essential oil or dried flowers, lavender can be incorporated into a warm bath or used as a room spray to create a peaceful ambiance.

Another powerful herb for calming the nervous system is lemon balm. This herb is known for its ability to reduce restlessness and promote a sense of calm. Lemon balm tea can be enjoyed throughout the day to help ease tension and anxiety. Additionally, passionflower is a well-known herb for its relaxing properties. It helps to calm both the mind and body, making it an excellent choice for those experiencing high levels of stress.

When it comes to relaxation, valerian root is a herb that cannot be overlooked. Valerian has been used for centuries as a natural sleep aid and anxiety reducer. Its sedative effects make it an excellent choice for those struggling with insomnia or restlessness.

To fully reap the benefits of these herbs, it is important to explore different methods of preparation. Herbal teas, tinctures, and essential oils are all effective ways to incorporate these herbs into your self-care routine. Experiment with different combinations and find what works best for you.

In conclusion, herbs offer a natural and effective way to promote relaxation and calm the nervous system. Chamomile, lavender, lemon balm, passionflower, and valerian root are just a few examples of herbs that can help reduce stress and anxiety. By incorporating these herbs into our daily routine, we can create a peaceful and nurturing environment for our overall well-being.

Adaptogenic Herbs for Balancing Stress Response

In today's fast-paced and demanding world, stress and anxiety have become a common part of our lives. As individuals interested in self-care with homeopathy, it is essential to explore natural remedies that can help us find balance and relieve these burdensome conditions. One powerful solution lies in the realm of adaptogenic herbs.

The Power of Nature: Essential Oils, Herbs, and Homeopathy for Stress and Anxiety Relief

Adaptogens are a class of herbs that have been used for centuries in traditional medicine systems like Ayurveda and Traditional Chinese Medicine (TCM). These herbs possess unique properties that help our bodies adapt to the physical, mental, and emotional stressors we encounter daily. They work by regulating the stress response system and promoting a state of homeostasis.

One of the most well-known adaptogenic herbs is Ashwagandha. Originating from India, this herb has gained popularity for its ability to reduce cortisol levels, the stress hormone, and promote a sense of calm and relaxation. Ashwagandha is often consumed as a supplement or in the form of a tea, and it can be an excellent addition to your self-care routine.

Another powerful adaptogen is Rhodiola Rosea, native to the cold regions of Europe and Asia. This herb has been used for centuries to combat fatigue, enhance mental performance, and reduce stress-related symptoms. Rhodiola Rosea is often recommended for those experiencing burnout or struggling with focus and concentration. It can be consumed in the form of a capsule or as a tincture.

Holy Basil, or Tulsi, is another adaptogenic herb worth exploring. Widely used in Ayurveda, Holy Basil is known for its calming properties and ability to support the adrenal glands. It helps balance stress hormones and promotes emotional well-being. Holy Basil can be enjoyed as a tea or taken as a supplement.

When it comes to utilizing these adaptogenic herbs, it is crucial to consult with a qualified homeopathic practitioner or herbalist. They can guide you on the appropriate dosage and help you choose the right herb based on your specific needs.

In conclusion, adaptogenic herbs offer a natural and effective approach to balance our stress response system and promote overall well-being. Incorporating herbs like Ashwagandha, Rhodiola Rosea, and Holy Basil into our self-care routines can significantly contribute to stress and anxiety relief. However, it is important to remember that everyone's body is unique, and it is always advisable to seek professional guidance when using herbs as part of your homeopathic self-care journey.

Herbal Supplements and Tinctures for Anxiety Relief

In our modernized world of today, stress and anxiety have become all too common. The constant demands of work, family, and personal life can leave us feeling overwhelmed and mentally exhausted. However, there is a natural and effective way to find relief from these daily struggles – through the power of herbal supplements and tinctures.

Herbs have been used for centuries to promote relaxation, calmness, and overall well-being. In this subchapter, we will explore the various herbal remedies that can be utilized for anxiety relief. Whether you are new to the world of herbal medicine or a seasoned practitioner, these natural alternatives can offer you the support you need to find inner peace and tranquility.

One of the most well-known herbs for anxiety relief is chamomile. This gentle flower has a long history of soothing nerves and promoting relaxation. Whether consumed as a tea or taken in tincture form, chamomile can help calm the mind and ease tension. Another popular herb is lavender, renowned for its calming scent. Lavender essential oil, when diffused or applied topically, can provide a sense of calm and help alleviate anxiety symptoms.

Additionally, passionflower has been used for centuries as a natural remedy for anxiety. This herb works by increasing levels of gamma-aminobutyric acid (GABA) in the brain, a neurotransmitter that helps regulate anxiety. Passionflower can be consumed as a tea or taken in tincture form.

Other notable herbs for anxiety relief include lemon balm, valerian root, and ashwagandha. Lemon balm has been shown to reduce anxiety and improve mood, while valerian root is known for its sedative properties, promoting better sleep and relaxation. Ashwagandha, an adaptogenic herb, helps the body adapt to stress and reduces anxiety symptoms.

When utilizing herbal supplements and tinctures, it's important to consult with a qualified herbalist or homeopath to determine the most appropriate dosage and duration of use. Everyone's body is unique, and what works for one person may not work for another.

In conclusion, the power of nature offers us a vast array of herbal remedies to combat stress and anxiety. By incorporating these natural alternatives into our self-care routine, we can find relief and support our overall well-being. Whether it's chamomile tea before bed or lavender oil in a diffuser, the gentle strength of these herbs can help us restore balance and find tranquility in our hectic lives.

Chapter 5: Introduction to Homeopathy

Understanding Homeopathy and Its Principles

The Power of Nature: Essential Oils, Herbs, and Homeopathy for Stress and Anxiety Relief

Homeopathy is a natural healing system that has been used for centuries to promote overall health and well-being. It is based on the principle of "like cures like," which means that a substance that can cause symptoms in a healthy person can be used to treat similar symptoms in a sick person. This subchapter aims to provide a comprehensive understanding of homeopathy and its key principles for individuals interested in self-care with homeopathy.

Homeopathy operates on the belief that the body has the inherent ability to heal itself. It stimulates this natural healing process by using highly diluted substances derived from plants, minerals, and animals. These substances are prepared through a process called potentization, which involves dilution and succussion (vigorous shaking). The more dilute the remedy, the more potent and powerful it becomes.

One of the fundamental principles of homeopathy is individualization. Homeopathic remedies are prescribed based on the unique symptoms and characteristics of each person. A homeopath carefully considers the physical, mental, and emotional aspects of an individual to determine the most suitable remedy. This personalized approach ensures that the treatment is tailored to the person's specific needs.

Another important principle of homeopathy is the concept of the vital force or life force. Homeopaths believe that the vital force is responsible for maintaining the body's balance and harmony. When this vital force is disrupted or imbalanced, it can lead to physical or emotional symptoms. Homeopathic remedies work by stimulating the vital force to restore balance and promote healing.

Homeopathy also emphasizes the importance of the minimum dose. Remedies are highly diluted to minimize any potential side effects. This makes homeopathy safe and suitable for people of all ages, including infants, pregnant women, and the elderly. It is a gentle and non-invasive approach to healing.

In this subchapter, we will explore the principles and philosophy of homeopathy, including the concepts of like cures like, individualization, the vital force, and the minimum dose. We will also discuss how homeopathy can be used to address stress and anxiety, in combination with essential oils and herbs. By understanding the principles of homeopathy, individuals can empower themselves to take control of their health and well-being naturally.

Whether you are new to homeopathy or have some experience with it, this subchapter will provide you with valuable insights and practical tips on how to incorporate homeopathy into your self-care routine.

How Homeopathy Works for Stress and Anxiety

In our current lifestyles, stress and anxiety have become common ailments that affect millions of individuals. Many people are now turning to alternative forms of medicine, such as homeopathy, to find relief from these conditions. This subchapter will explore how homeopathy works for stress and anxiety and how it can be utilized effectively in self-care routines.

The Power of Nature: Essential Oils, Herbs, and Homeopathy for Stress and Anxiety Relief

Homeopathy is a holistic system of medicine that focuses on stimulating the body's natural ability to heal itself. It is based on the principle of "like cures like," which means that a substance that can cause symptoms in a healthy person can be used to treat similar symptoms in an ailing person. Homeopathic remedies are made from natural substances, such as plants, minerals, or animal products, and are highly diluted to activate the body's healing response without causing any harm.

When it comes to stress and anxiety relief, homeopathy offers a gentle and non-invasive approach. Homeopathic remedies aim to address the underlying causes of stress and anxiety rather than simply masking the symptoms. By restoring balance to the body and mind, homeopathy helps individuals achieve a state of calm and relaxation.

There are various homeopathic remedies that can be used for different types of stress and anxiety. For instance, Aconitum napellus is often recommended for acute anxiety and panic attacks, while Argentum nitricum is useful for anticipatory anxiety. Ignatia amara is commonly used for grief-related anxiety, and Natrum muriaticum is beneficial for anxiety associated with suppressed emotions.

In this subchapter, we will delve into the specific homeopathic remedies that are effective for stress and anxiety relief. We will explore their individual properties, recommended dosages, and how to choose the right remedy based on individual symptoms and constitution. Additionally, we will discuss the importance of consulting with a qualified homeopathic practitioner to ensure the most appropriate remedy is selected.

Furthermore, this subchapter will provide practical tips on incorporating homeopathy into daily self-care routines. We will discuss the benefits of combining homeopathic remedies with essential oils and herbs known for their calming and soothing properties. By harnessing the power of nature, individuals can create personalized stress and anxiety relief regimens that promote overall well-being.

Whether you are new to homeopathy or have already experienced its benefits, this subchapter will serve as a comprehensive guide to utilizing homeopathy for stress and anxiety relief. By understanding how homeopathy works and learning how to incorporate it into your self-care routine, you can take control of your mental and emotional well-being naturally and effectively.

Selecting the Right Homeopathic Remedies

When it comes to managing stress and anxiety, homeopathy is a powerful tool that can help restore balance and promote overall well-being. With the vast array of homeopathic remedies available, it is crucial to understand how to select the right ones for your individual needs. This subchapter will guide individuals interested in self-care with homeopathy, focusing on the selection process of appropriate remedies.

Before diving into the specifics, it is important to note that homeopathy treats the individual as a whole, taking into account their physical, emotional, and mental symptoms. This holistic approach makes it essential to carefully evaluate your symptoms and choose remedies that match your unique state of being.

To begin, it is recommended to consult with a qualified homeopath who can assess your symptoms and recommend appropriate remedies. However, for those who prefer self-care, there are a few key considerations to keep in mind when selecting homeopathic remedies.

Firstly, it is crucial to identify the specific symptoms you are experiencing. Are you feeling restless, agitated, or overwhelmed? Or are you experiencing physical symptoms such as headaches, muscle tension, or digestive issues? By pinpointing your symptoms, you can narrow down the remedies that are most likely to address your concerns.

Secondly, it is important to research and understand the properties and indications of various homeopathic remedies. Each remedy has its own unique set of characteristics and is tailored to address specific symptoms. For instance, if you are feeling anxious with a racing mind, remedies like Argentum nitricum or Gelsemium may be beneficial. On the other hand, if you are experiencing physical symptoms like palpitations or trembling, remedies such as Aconite or Ignatia might be more suitable.

Lastly, it is crucial to start with a low potency and observe the effects of the remedy. Homeopathic remedies are typically available in various potencies, and it is advisable to begin with a lower potency (such as 6C or 30C) to gauge the response. If needed, the potency can be adjusted based on the individual's feedback.

Remember, homeopathy is a gentle and natural approach to healing, but it may take time and experimentation to find the remedies that work best for you. It is essential to be patient and persistent in your self-care journey.

By carefully evaluating your symptoms, researching remedies, and starting with a low potency, you can confidently select the right homeopathic remedies to manage stress and anxiety. Harness the power of nature and embark on your path to holistic well-being with homeopathy.

Dosage and Administration of Homeopathic Remedies

The Power of Nature: Essential Oils, Herbs, and Homeopathy for Stress and Anxiety Relief

Homeopathy is a natural form of medicine that utilizes diluted substances to stimulate the body's own healing abilities. When it comes to dosage and administration of homeopathic remedies, it is crucial to understand the principles behind this unique approach. In this subchapter, we will explore the guidelines for effectively utilizing homeopathic remedies for stress and anxiety relief.

Homeopathic remedies are available in various forms, including pellets, tablets, liquid solutions, and creams. The dosage and administration of these remedies depend on several factors, including the severity of symptoms, individual sensitivity, and the specific remedy being used. It is always recommended to consult a qualified homeopathic practitioner for personalized advice, especially if you are new to homeopathy.

One of the fundamental principles of homeopathy is the concept of individualization. This means that the remedy chosen should match the unique symptoms and characteristics of the individual. Homeopathic remedies are selected based on a holistic understanding of the person's mental, emotional, and physical state. Therefore, it is essential to carefully observe and describe your symptoms to find the most suitable remedy.

In terms of dosage, homeopathic remedies are typically administered in small amounts to trigger the body's self-healing response. This is achieved through a process called potentization, where the original substance is diluted and succussed (shaken vigorously). The potency of a remedy is indicated by a number and letter combination, such as 6X or 30C. The higher the number, the greater the dilution and potency.

When using homeopathic remedies for stress and anxiety relief, it is generally recommended to start with a low potency, such as 6X or 6C. Take a single dose and observe the response. If there is no change, the remedy may need to be repeated at regular intervals, such as every few hours or once a day. However, if symptoms worsen or new symptoms arise, it is advisable to stop taking the remedy and consult a professional homeopath.

It is important to note that homeopathic remedies should be taken on a clean palate, away from food, beverages, and strong flavors. Avoid brushing your teeth or using strong mouthwash before or after taking the remedy, as these may interfere with its effectiveness.

In conclusion, homeopathic remedies offer a natural and holistic approach to stress and anxiety relief. By understanding the principles of dosage and administration, individuals interested in self-care with homeopathy can effectively utilize these remedies. Remember to consult a qualified homeopathic practitioner for personalized advice and always follow the recommended guidelines to ensure safe and effective results.

Chapter 6: Homeopathic Remedies for Stress and Anxiety Relief

Ignatia Amara: Healing Emotional Grief and Loss

The Power of Nature: Essential Oils, Herbs, and Homeopathy for Stress and Anxiety Relief

In the realm of homeopathy, Ignatia Amara is a powerful remedy that offers profound healing for emotional grief and loss. Derived from the seeds of the St. Ignatius bean, this natural remedy has been used for centuries to support individuals experiencing deep sorrow, heartbreak, and emotional upheaval. In this subchapter, we will explore the therapeutic benefits of Ignatia Amara and how it can be effectively utilized to heal emotional wounds.

Grief and loss are universal experiences that can be incredibly challenging to navigate. Whether it's the loss of a loved one, the end of a relationship, or the disappointment of unfulfilled dreams, these emotional upheavals can leave us feeling overwhelmed, vulnerable, and disconnected from ourselves. Ignatia Amara offers solace and support during these difficult times, gently guiding us towards healing and emotional well-being.

One of the key features of Ignatia Amara is its ability to address the complex emotions associated with grief and loss. It can help individuals who experience sudden mood swings, intense sadness, or emotional outbursts. By acting on the nervous system, Ignatia Amara helps to stabilize and balance emotions, allowing for a healthier processing of grief.

Furthermore, Ignatia Amara can provide relief from physical symptoms that often accompany emotional distress. Individuals experiencing headaches, insomnia, and digestive disturbances due to grief can find relief through this remedy. By addressing both the emotional and physical aspects of grief, Ignatia Amara offers comprehensive support for holistic healing.

In this subchapter, you will discover practical ways to incorporate Ignatia Amara into your self-care routine. Whether it's using Ignatia Amara essential oil in a diffuser, preparing a herbal tea infusion, or taking Ignatia Amara homeopathic pellets, there are various methods to harness its healing properties. We will provide you with step-by-step instructions and dosage guidelines, ensuring that you can safely and effectively utilize this remedy.

By incorporating Ignatia Amara into your self-care routine, you can embark on a journey of emotional healing and find solace in the midst of grief and loss. This subchapter aims to empower individuals interested in self-care with homeopathy, offering a comprehensive guide to utilizing essential oils, herbs, and homeopathy for stress and anxiety relief. By embracing the power of nature's remedies, you can tap into your inner strength, find balance, and restore emotional well-being.

Arsenicum Album: Easing Restlessness and Panic

When it comes to finding natural remedies for stress and anxiety, homeopathy offers a wide range of options. Among the many effective remedies, Arsenicum Album stands out for its ability to ease restlessness and panic. This subchapter explores the potential of Arsenicum Album in helping individuals find relief from these distressing symptoms.

Arsenicum Album is a homeopathic remedy derived from the mineral arsenic. While arsenic may seem like an unlikely source of healing, when prepared in a highly diluted form through the homeopathic process, it becomes a potent remedy for various ailments. In the case of stress and anxiety, Arsenicum Album has gained popularity for its ability to calm the mind and restore a sense of tranquility.

The Power of Nature: Essential Oils, Herbs, and Homeopathy for Stress and Anxiety Relief

Restlessness is a common symptom experienced by individuals dealing with stress and anxiety. They often find it challenging to sit still or relax, constantly feeling the need to be on the move. Arsenicum Album addresses this restlessness by promoting a sense of serenity and grounding. It helps individuals feel more centered and at ease, allowing them to find comfort in stillness.

Panic attacks can be incredibly debilitating, causing intense fear and a sense of impending doom. Arsenicum Album has shown promise in alleviating these panic symptoms. It helps to reduce the intensity and frequency of panic attacks, allowing individuals to regain control over their emotions. By calming the mind and soothing the nervous system, Arsenicum Album provides much-needed relief during moments of distress.

To utilize Arsenicum Album effectively, it is recommended to consult with a qualified homeopath who can prescribe the appropriate dosage and potency based on individual symptoms and needs. Homeopathy considers the unique characteristics of each person, tailoring the remedy to their specific mental, emotional, and physical state.

In addition to Arsenicum Album, this book explores other essential oils, herbs, and homeopathic remedies that can be utilized for stress and anxiety relief. By understanding the power of nature and incorporating these natural remedies into your self-care routine, you can find a holistic approach to managing stress and anxiety.

Remember, self-care is essential, and homeopathy provides a gentle and effective way to support your well-being. By exploring the potential of Arsenicum Album and other remedies, you can take control of your stress and anxiety, finding balance and peace in your life.

Gelsemium: Alleviating Performance Anxiety and Nervousness

With our current busy and stressful lifestyles, anxiety has become an all too common issue. Whether it's the pressure of a big presentation at work, a nerve-wracking performance on stage, or simply dealing with the demands of everyday life, it's important to find effective ways to alleviate these feelings and regain a sense of calm. One natural remedy that has gained recognition for its ability to combat performance anxiety and nervousness is Gelsemium.

Gelsemium, a flowering plant native to North America and Asia, has been used in homeopathy for centuries. It is known for its calming and soothing properties, making it an ideal choice for individuals seeking relief from stress and anxiety. This powerful herb can be used in various forms, including essential oils, tinctures, and teas, making it easily accessible to those interested in self-care with homeopathy.

When it comes to performance anxiety, Gelsemium is particularly effective. Many people experience heightened nervousness and anxiety before an important event, such as a public speaking engagement or a musical performance. Gelsemium can help alleviate these symptoms by reducing muscle tension, promoting relaxation, and calming the mind. It works by targeting the nervous system, helping to restore balance and tranquility.

To utilize Gelsemium for stress and anxiety relief, there are several options available. Gelsemium essential oil can be diffused in a room or added to a carrier oil for topical application. Inhaling the aroma of Gelsemium can have an immediate calming effect, allowing you to feel more centered and focused. Additionally, Gelsemium tinctures and teas can be consumed to promote a sense of relaxation and ease anxiety symptoms.

It's important to note that while Gelsemium is generally safe for most individuals, it is always advisable to consult with a qualified homeopathic practitioner before using any new remedy. They can provide personalized guidance and ensure that Gelsemium is the right choice for your specific needs.

In conclusion, Gelsemium is a powerful natural remedy that can help alleviate performance anxiety and nervousness. By incorporating Gelsemium into your self-care routine, you can experience the calming and soothing benefits of this remarkable herb. Take control of your stress and anxiety with the power of nature and embrace a more balanced and fulfilling life.

Aconitum Napellus: Calming Acute Anxiety and Panic Attacks

When it comes to finding natural remedies for stress and anxiety relief, Aconitum Napellus is a homeopathic remedy that should not be overlooked. Derived from the flowering plant commonly known as monkshood, Aconitum Napellus has been used for centuries to alleviate acute anxiety and panic attacks.

If you are an individual interested in self-care with homeopathy, understanding the benefits and usage of Aconitum Napellus can be incredibly beneficial. This subchapter aims to shed light on this powerful remedy and how it can be utilized effectively to bring about calmness during moments of intense anxiety or panic.

Aconitum Napellus works by targeting the nervous system, soothing and calming it during times of distress. It is particularly useful when anxiety or panic attacks arise suddenly, often triggered by a specific event or situation. This remedy is known to provide rapid relief, helping to reduce feelings of fear, restlessness, and trembling.

The Power of Nature: Essential Oils, Herbs, and Homeopathy for Stress and Anxiety Relief

To use Aconitum Napellus, it is essential to consult with a qualified homeopathic practitioner to determine the correct dosage and potency for your specific needs. Homeopathy is an individualized form of medicine, and the right dosage will vary from person to person. By working closely with a professional, you can ensure that you are taking the remedy in the most effective and safe manner.

When acute anxiety or panic strikes, taking Aconitum Napellus in the recommended dosage can help bring about a sense of calmness and alleviate the intensity of symptoms. It can be taken orally in the form of pellets or liquid, allowing for quick absorption into the system.

It is important to note that while Aconitum Napellus can provide significant relief for acute anxiety and panic attacks, it should not replace professional medical care for chronic or severe cases. If you are experiencing ongoing anxiety or panic disorder, it is crucial to seek the guidance of a healthcare professional who can provide a comprehensive treatment plan.

In conclusion, Aconitum Napellus is a valuable homeopathic remedy that can effectively calm acute anxiety and panic attacks. By utilizing this natural remedy, individuals interested in self-care with homeopathy can find relief during moments of intense distress. However, it is essential to consult with a homeopathic practitioner to ensure the correct dosage and potency for your specific needs. Remember, self-care is a journey, and finding the right tools to manage stress and anxiety is a vital step towards overall well-being.

Lycopodium Clavatum: Boosting Confidence and Reducing Anxiety

The Power of Nature: Essential Oils, Herbs, and Homeopathy for Stress and Anxiety Relief

In the quest for natural remedies to combat stress and anxiety, homeopathy has emerged as a powerful tool. Among the various remedies available, Lycopodium Clavatum has gained significant popularity for its ability to boost confidence and reduce anxiety. This subchapter delves into the incredible potential of Lycopodium Clavatum and how it can be harnessed to promote self-care and well-being.

Lycopodium Clavatum, commonly known as Club Moss, is a unique herb that has been used for centuries in homeopathy to address a range of physical and emotional ailments. When it comes to anxiety, Lycopodium Clavatum is highly regarded for its profound impact on confidence levels. Many individuals who struggle with anxiety often find themselves plagued by self-doubt and a lack of self-assurance. Lycopodium Clavatum works by restoring faith in one's abilities and promoting a sense of inner strength and resilience.

One of the key benefits of Lycopodium Clavatum is its calming effect on the nervous system. Anxiety often manifests as restlessness, racing thoughts, and an overwhelming sense of unease. By gently calming the nervous system, Lycopodium Clavatum can help individuals find a sense of peace and tranquility. This natural remedy has been known to alleviate symptoms such as irritability, sleep disturbances, and digestive issues that often accompany anxiety.

To harness the power of Lycopodium Clavatum, it is recommended to consult with a qualified homeopath who can guide you through the process. Homeopathic remedies are tailored to the individual's unique symptoms and constitution, ensuring the most effective and personalized treatment.

In addition to homeopathic remedies, Lycopodium Clavatum can also be utilized in the form of essential oils and herbal preparations. Aromatherapy with Lycopodium Clavatum essential oil can create a soothing and calming environment, promoting relaxation and reducing anxiety symptoms. Herbal preparations such as teas or tinctures can be used to support the body's natural healing process and enhance overall well-being.

By incorporating Lycopodium Clavatum into your self-care routine, you can experience the profound benefits of this powerful remedy. Whether you choose to explore homeopathic remedies or incorporate essential oils and herbs into your daily life, Lycopodium Clavatum offers a natural and holistic approach to reducing anxiety and boosting confidence. Embrace the power of nature and empower yourself on your journey towards stress and anxiety relief.

Chapter 7: Creating a Self-Care Routine with Essential Oils, Herbs, and Homeopathy

Designing a Stress-Relieving Environment

Creating a stress-free environment is crucial for maintaining overall well-being and mental health. Whether you are dealing with everyday stressors or battling anxiety, designing a stress-relieving environment can significantly improve your quality of life. In this subchapter, we will explore how to utilize essential oils and herbs to create a soothing and calming atmosphere that promotes relaxation and reduces stress and anxiety.

The Power of Nature: Essential Oils, Herbs, and Homeopathy for Stress and Anxiety Relief

Essential oils have been used for centuries to alleviate stress and anxiety. Their aromatic properties can positively impact our mood and emotions, helping us to unwind and find inner peace. Lavender, for example, is well-known for its calming effects and can be diffused in your living space to create a serene ambiance. Similarly, bergamot and chamomile are also great options for promoting relaxation and reducing anxiety.

In addition to essential oils, incorporating herbs into your stress-relieving environment can enhance its effectiveness. Herbs like valerian root and passionflower have been traditionally used to ease anxiety and promote better sleep. These herbs can be consumed as teas or tinctures, or even used in a sachet placed under your pillow to aid in relaxation and stress relief.

When designing your stress-relieving environment, consider the following tips:

1. Declutter: A cluttered space can increase stress levels. Clear out unnecessary items and create an organized and peaceful atmosphere.

2. Natural Light: Allow as much natural light as possible into your space. Sunlight can boost mood and reduce anxiety.

3. Nature-Inspired Decor: Incorporate elements of nature into your environment. Plants, soothing colors, and natural materials can create a calming ambiance.

4. Aromatherapy: Utilize essential oils through diffusers, room sprays, or even by adding a few drops to a warm bath. Experiment with different scents to find what works best for you.

5. Relaxation Zones: Designate specific areas for relaxation, such as a cozy reading nook or a meditation corner. These spaces can help you escape from the daily stressors and unwind.

By incorporating these elements into your environment, you can create a stress-relieving sanctuary that supports your self-care journey. Remember, everyone is unique, so don't hesitate to experiment and find what works best for you. With the power of essential oils, herbs, and homeopathy, you can alleviate stress and anxiety, enhance your overall well-being, and enjoy a more balanced and peaceful life.

Daily Rituals for Balancing Stress and Anxiety

In our fast-paced modern world, it is not uncommon to experience stress and anxiety on a daily basis. The demands of work, family, and personal life can easily take a toll on our mental and emotional well-being. However, there are simple and effective daily rituals that can help us find balance and relief from the pressures of life.

One powerful tool in managing stress and anxiety is the use of essential oils. These concentrated plant extracts have been used for centuries to promote relaxation and calmness. Incorporating essential oils into your daily routine can have a profound impact on your overall well-being. For instance, you can start your day by diffusing lavender oil, known for its soothing properties, to create a calm and peaceful atmosphere. Inhaling the aroma of lavender can help reduce feelings of stress and anxiety, setting a positive tone for the day.

The Power of Nature: Essential Oils, Herbs, and Homeopathy for Stress and Anxiety Relief

Another way to utilize essential oils is through topical application. You can create a personalized blend by combining a few drops of your favorite calming oils, such as chamomile, bergamot, or ylang-ylang, with a carrier oil like sweet almond or jojoba. Gently massaging this blend onto your temples, wrists, or the back of your neck can provide instant relief from tension and promote relaxation.

In addition to essential oils, incorporating herbs into your daily routine can also be beneficial for stress and anxiety relief. Herbal teas, such as chamomile, lemon balm, or passionflower, can have a calming effect on the nervous system when enjoyed throughout the day. Taking the time to sit down and savor a cup of herbal tea can be a meditative practice that helps shift your focus away from stressors and promotes a sense of calm.

Homeopathy, a natural system of medicine, offers a wide range of remedies for managing stress and anxiety. Consultation with a qualified homeopath can help identify the most suitable remedy for your individual needs. Taking a daily dose of the recommended homeopathic remedy can support your body's natural ability to cope with stress and promote emotional balance.

In conclusion, incorporating daily rituals into your life can make a significant difference in managing stress and anxiety. Utilizing the power of nature through essential oils, herbs, and homeopathy can provide effective relief and promote overall well-being. By taking the time to prioritize self-care and implementing these rituals, individuals interested in homeopathy can find a natural and holistic approach to find balance and tranquility in their daily lives.

Incorporating Essential Oils into Your Self-Care Routine

The Power of Nature: Essential Oils, Herbs, and Homeopathy for Stress and Anxiety Relief

Self-care is essential for maintaining our overall well-being, especially in today's fast-paced and stressful world. If you are someone who is interested in exploring natural remedies for stress and anxiety relief, incorporating essential oils into your self-care routine can be a game-changer. In this subchapter, we will discuss how to utilize essential oils and herbs to enhance your self-care practices and promote a sense of calm and relaxation.

Essential oils have been used for centuries for their therapeutic properties. They are derived from plants and contain powerful compounds that can positively impact our physical and emotional health. When used correctly, essential oils can help reduce stress, anxiety, and promote a sense of well-being.

One of the most effective ways to incorporate essential oils into your self-care routine is through aromatherapy. Aromatherapy involves using essential oils either through inhalation or topical application. By diffusing essential oils in your home or office, you can create an environment that promotes relaxation and reduces stress. Lavender, chamomile, and bergamot are excellent choices for calming and soothing effects.

Another way to enjoy the benefits of essential oils is by adding them to your bath. Adding a few drops of essential oils such as ylang-ylang or clary sage to your bathwater can help you unwind and release tension. You can also create your own massage oil by diluting essential oils with a carrier oil like coconut or jojoba oil. Massaging this blend onto your body can help relieve muscle tension and promote relaxation.

The Power of Nature: Essential Oils, Herbs, and Homeopathy for Stress and Anxiety Relief

In addition to essential oils, herbs can also play a vital role in your self-care routine. Herbal teas made from chamomile, lemon balm, or passionflower can help calm the mind and promote restful sleep. Adding herbs like valerian root or ashwagandha to your daily supplement routine can also help reduce anxiety and promote a sense of calm.

When incorporating essential oils and herbs into your self-care routine, it's important to choose high-quality products and follow proper usage guidelines. Always dilute essential oils before applying them to your skin, and conduct a patch test to check for any allergies or sensitivities. If you have any underlying health conditions or are taking medication, it's best to consult with a qualified healthcare practitioner before using essential oils or herbs.

By incorporating essential oils and herbs into your self-care routine, you can harness the power of nature to reduce stress and anxiety, promote relaxation, and enhance your overall well-being. Experiment with different oils and herbs to find what works best for you, and remember to prioritize self-care as an essential part of your daily routine.

Utilizing Herbs for Daily Wellness

Many individuals are seeking natural remedies to support their mental and emotional well-being. One powerful approach to self-care is incorporating herbs into our daily routines. In this subchapter, we will explore the benefits of utilizing herbs for daily wellness and how they can be effectively used to alleviate stress and anxiety.

The Power of Nature: Essential Oils, Herbs, and Homeopathy for Stress and Anxiety Relief

Herbs have been used for centuries in various cultures as natural remedies for a wide range of ailments. When it comes to stress and anxiety relief, certain herbs possess unique properties that can help soothe the mind and promote relaxation. One such herb is chamomile, known for its calming effects. Whether enjoyed as a warm cup of tea or used in essential oil form, chamomile can help ease tension and promote a restful night's sleep.

Another herb that has gained popularity in recent years is lavender. With its delightful fragrance and soothing properties, lavender is a go-to herb for stress relief. Its essential oil can be diffused in the air, applied topically, or added to a warm bath to create a calming environment and promote relaxation.

In addition to chamomile and lavender, there are several other herbs that can be incorporated into our daily routines for stress and anxiety relief. Lemon balm, passionflower, and valerian root are all known for their calming effects on the nervous system. These herbs can be consumed as teas, tinctures, or taken as supplements in consultation with a qualified healthcare professional.

When utilizing herbs for daily wellness, it's important to remember that everyone's response may vary. It may be helpful to start with small doses and gradually increase as needed, while closely monitoring how your body and mind respond. Additionally, it's crucial to consult with a knowledgeable healthcare practitioner, particularly if you have any underlying health conditions or are taking medications.

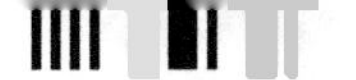

Incorporating herbs into our daily routines is a gentle and natural way to support our mental and emotional well-being. By harnessing the power of nature, we can find relief from stress and anxiety and promote a sense of peace and balance in our lives. Remember, self-care is essential, and herbs can be a valuable tool in our journey towards overall wellness.

Integrating Homeopathic Remedies for Long-Term Relief

When it comes to finding long-term relief from stress and anxiety, homeopathic remedies can be a fantastic addition to your self-care routine. Homeopathy is a holistic approach to healing that uses highly diluted substances derived from plants, minerals, and other natural sources to stimulate the body's natural healing abilities. In this subchapter, we will explore how you can integrate homeopathic remedies into your daily life to find lasting relief from stress and anxiety.

One of the great benefits of homeopathy is its ability to address the underlying causes of stress and anxiety, rather than just treating the symptoms. Homeopathic remedies are tailored to each individual's unique symptoms and constitution, making them a personalized and effective solution. By addressing the root causes of your stress and anxiety, homeopathy can help you achieve long-term relief.

There are several key homeopathic remedies that are particularly effective in managing stress and anxiety. For example, if you experience restlessness, irritability, and anxiety that is aggravated by noise or light, Ignatia Amara may be a suitable remedy for you. On the other hand, if you have anticipatory anxiety, a fear of failure, and a tendency to overwork, Argentum Nitricum might be a better fit.

To integrate homeopathic remedies into your self-care routine, it is important to consult with a qualified homeopath who can prescribe the appropriate remedies for your specific needs. They will take into account your individual symptoms, medical history, and overall constitution to create a personalized treatment plan.

In addition to taking homeopathic remedies, there are other ways you can support your body's natural healing abilities. Essential oils and herbs can complement homeopathy by promoting relaxation and reducing stress. Lavender essential oil, for instance, is known for its calming properties, while herbs like chamomile and lemon balm can help soothe anxiety and promote a sense of peace.

Remember, homeopathic remedies work best when integrated into a holistic approach to wellness. Alongside taking remedies and incorporating essential oils and herbs, it is essential to prioritize self-care practices such as regular exercise, a nutritious diet, and mindfulness activities like meditation or yoga.

By integrating homeopathic remedies into your self-care routine, you can find long-term relief from stress and anxiety. Embrace the power of nature and discover how homeopathy, essential oils, and herbs can support your journey towards a more balanced and serene life.

Chapter 8: Additional Techniques for Stress and Anxiety Management

Mindfulness and Meditation Practices

The Power of Nature: Essential Oils, Herbs, and Homeopathy for Stress and Anxiety Relief

In today's stress-filled world, finding effective ways to manage your stress and anxiety is essential for maintaining overall well-being. While essential oils and herbs can certainly play a significant role in stress relief, incorporating mindfulness and meditation practices into your self-care routine can further enhance their benefits. In this subchapter, we will explore how mindfulness and meditation can complement the use of essential oils and herbs for stress and anxiety relief.

Mindfulness is the practice of being fully present and aware of the present moment without judgment. By cultivating mindfulness, we can develop a deeper understanding of our thoughts, feelings, and bodily sensations, allowing us to respond to stressors in a more calm and centered manner. When combined with the therapeutic properties of essential oils and herbs, mindfulness can amplify their effects, promoting a state of relaxation and tranquility.

Meditation, on the other hand, involves intentionally focusing the mind and achieving a heightened sense of awareness and inner peace. Regular meditation practice has been shown to reduce stress, anxiety, and even improve sleep quality. When used alongside essential oils and herbs, meditation can create a synergistic effect, helping to alleviate stress and anxiety on a profound level.

To incorporate mindfulness and meditation into your stress relief routine, begin by finding a quiet and comfortable space where you can relax without distractions. Close your eyes, take a few deep breaths, and allow your mind to settle. You can enhance your meditation practice by diffusing calming essential oils such as lavender or chamomile, or by brewing a cup of herbal tea like passionflower or lemon balm.

As you become more adept at mindfulness and meditation, you can start exploring guided meditation apps or online resources tailored specifically for stress and anxiety relief. These resources often incorporate visualization techniques and affirmations, which, when combined with the therapeutic properties of essential oils and herbs, can further deepen your relaxation experience.

In conclusion, by incorporating mindfulness and meditation practices into your self-care routine, you can enhance the stress-relieving benefits of essential oils and herbs. Mindfulness allows you to be fully present and aware, while meditation helps to cultivate inner peace and tranquility. Together, these practices create a powerful synergy that can support you on your journey towards optimal well-being. So, take a moment to pause, breathe, and embrace the power of mindfulness and meditation in your stress and anxiety relief journey.

Breathing Exercises for Relaxation

In the fast-paced world we live in today, stress and anxiety have become all too common. The constant demands of work, family, and personal life can take a toll on our mental and physical well-being. However, there are natural and effective ways to combat stress and anxiety, and one of the most powerful tools at our disposal is our breath. By learning and practicing simple breathing exercises, we can tap into the power of nature and find relaxation and calm amidst the chaos.

Breathing exercises have been used for centuries in various healing practices, including homeopathy, to promote relaxation and reduce stress. These exercises work by activating the body's natural relaxation response, which helps to counteract the effects of the fight-or-flight response triggered by stress. By focusing on our breath, we can slow down our heart rate, lower blood pressure, and induce a state of deep relaxation.

The Power of Nature: Essential Oils, Herbs, and Homeopathy for Stress and Anxiety Relief

One of the simplest and most effective breathing exercises for relaxation is deep belly breathing. To practice this exercise, find a quiet and comfortable space where you won't be disturbed. Sit or lie down in a relaxed position, and place one hand on your belly. Take a slow, deep breath in through your nose, allowing your belly to rise as you fill your lungs with air. Pause for a moment, and then exhale slowly through your mouth, feeling your belly fall. Repeat this process for several minutes, focusing on the sensation of your breath as it enters and leaves your body.

Another powerful breathing exercise is the 4-7-8 technique. This exercise involves inhaling for a count of four, holding your breath for a count of seven, and exhaling for a count of eight. This technique helps to regulate the breath and activate the body's relaxation response. Practice this exercise for a few minutes each day, preferably in a quiet and peaceful environment.

To enhance the benefits of these breathing exercises, you can incorporate the use of essential oils and herbs known for their calming properties. Lavender, chamomile, and bergamot essential oils can be diffused or applied topically to promote relaxation. Similarly, herbal teas such as chamomile, lemon balm, and passionflower can be enjoyed before or during your breathing exercises to enhance their soothing effects.

By incorporating breathing exercises into your daily routine and harnessing the power of nature through essential oils and herbs, you can effectively manage stress and anxiety in a natural and holistic way. Take the time to nurture yourself and prioritize self-care with these simple yet powerful techniques. Remember, the breath is always with you, ready to bring you back to a state of calm and peace.

Yoga and Movement for Stress Relief

The Power of Nature: Essential Oils, Herbs, and Homeopathy for Stress and Anxiety Relief

In this subchapter, we delve into the powerful combination of yoga and movement in alleviating stress and anxiety. As individuals interested in self-care with homeopathy, it is essential to recognize that stress affects not only our mental well-being but also our physical health. Incorporating yoga and movement practices into our daily routines can provide a holistic approach to managing stress and anxiety.

Yoga, an ancient practice originating from India, focuses on harmonizing the mind, body, and spirit. It combines physical postures, breathing exercises, and meditation to promote relaxation and inner peace. Numerous studies have shown that practicing yoga regularly can decrease stress hormones, lower blood pressure, and improve overall well-being.

When it comes to stress relief, specific yoga poses can target tension and anxiety directly. For example, the Child's Pose (Balasana) and the Corpse Pose (Savasana) can help calm the nervous system and induce deep relaxation. The Cat-Cow pose (Marjaryasana-Bitilasana) and the Standing Forward Bend (Uttanasana) can release built-up tension in the back and shoulders, areas prone to stress-related discomfort.

Movement, on the other hand, refers to any physical activity that engages the body and promotes flexibility, strength, and cardiovascular health. Engaging in regular movement not only helps reduce stress but also releases endorphins, the body's natural mood enhancers. This subchapter explores various types of movement, including dance, walking, jogging, and tai chi, each offering unique benefits for stress relief.

In addition to yoga and movement practices, we also explore how to enhance the stress-relieving effects by incorporating essential oils and herbs. Certain essential oils, such as lavender, chamomile, and bergamot, have calming properties and can be diffused, applied topically, or used for aromatherapy during yoga and movement sessions. Similarly, herbs like ashwagandha, lemon balm, and passionflower can be consumed as teas, tinctures, or supplements to promote relaxation and reduce anxiety.

By incorporating yoga and movement into our self-care routines and utilizing essential oils and herbs, we can create a powerful synergy for stress and anxiety relief. This subchapter provides practical tips, step-by-step guides, and expert advice on how to integrate these practices seamlessly into our lives. Remember, self-care is an ongoing journey, and by exploring the power of nature through yoga, movement, and natural remedies, we can find solace, balance, and peace in our daily lives.

Journaling and Expressive Arts Therapy

In the pursuit of self-care and holistic well-being, there is a growing recognition of the profound healing benefits of journaling and expressive arts therapy. These therapeutic practices offer individuals a creative outlet to explore their emotions, thoughts, and experiences, while also providing a means to alleviate stress and anxiety. This subchapter aims to delve into the transformative power of journaling and expressive arts therapy, specifically in conjunction with the use of essential oils, herbs, and homeopathy.

Journaling is a form of self-expression that allows individuals to reflect on their innermost thoughts and feelings. By putting pen to paper, one can release pent-up emotions, gain clarity, and develop a deeper understanding of oneself. Incorporating essential oils and herbs into the journaling process can enhance its therapeutic effects. Certain scents, such as lavender or chamomile, can promote relaxation and help reduce anxiety while writing. Similarly, herbal teas or tinctures like lemon balm or passionflower can be consumed before journaling to calm the mind and enhance focus.

Expressive arts therapy expands on the benefits of journaling by incorporating various art forms, including painting, drawing, collage, and even movement. This approach encourages individuals to explore their emotions and experiences through creative expression, allowing for a deeper exploration and release of stress and anxiety. Essential oils can be diffused in the therapy space to create a calming atmosphere, while herbal remedies, such as valerian or St. John's Wort, can be used to support emotional balance during the creative process.

By combining the power of journaling and expressive arts therapy with the therapeutic benefits of essential oils, herbs, and homeopathy, individuals can experience a profound transformation in their overall well-being. These practices provide a safe and nurturing space to explore and process emotions, reduce stress, and cultivate inner peace.

Whether you are new to journaling and expressive arts therapy or have dabbled in these practices before, this subchapter will guide you on how to integrate essential oils, herbs, and homeopathy into your self-care routine. It will offer tips, techniques, and creative exercises to help you tap into your inner wisdom and harness the healing potential of nature.

The Power of Nature: Essential Oils, Herbs, and Homeopathy for Stress and Anxiety Relief

Embark on this journey of self-discovery and self-care, and unlock the power of journaling and expressive arts therapy as essential tools for stress and anxiety relief. Your path to holistic well-being awaits you.

Seeking Professional Help and Support

In our journey toward holistic well-being, it is important to recognize that self-care goes beyond just utilizing essential oils and herbs. While these natural remedies can be incredibly powerful for stress and anxiety relief, there may be times when seeking professional help and support becomes necessary.

When it comes to managing stress and anxiety, it is crucial to remember that each individual's experience is unique. What works for one person may not work for another, and sometimes, deeper issues may be at play that require professional guidance. This is where the expertise of homeopaths and other healthcare professionals comes into play.

Homeopathy, as a complementary therapy, can be a fantastic tool for stress and anxiety relief. However, it is essential to consult a trained homeopath to ensure proper diagnosis and treatment. Homeopaths are skilled in understanding the underlying causes of stress and anxiety and can prescribe remedies tailored to your specific needs. They take into account not only your physical symptoms but also your emotional and mental well-being, providing a holistic approach to healing.

Additionally, seeking support from mental health professionals such as psychologists or therapists can be immensely beneficial. These professionals can help you explore the root causes of your stress and anxiety and provide you with effective coping strategies. They offer a safe space to express your feelings and emotions, allowing you to gain insights into yourself and develop healthier ways of managing stress.

Remember, there is no shame in seeking professional help. In fact, it is a sign of strength and self-awareness to recognize when you need support beyond what you can provide for yourself. Seeking professional help can accelerate your healing process and provide you with the tools to navigate life's challenges more effectively.

In conclusion, while essential oils and herbs are powerful allies in managing stress and anxiety, seeking professional help and support is sometimes necessary for a comprehensive approach to self-care. Homeopaths and mental health professionals can offer valuable insights, personalized treatment plans, and emotional support to help you on your journey toward holistic well-being. Don't hesitate to reach out to these experts and embrace the power of their guidance alongside the natural remedies you are already utilizing. Your mental and emotional health deserve the utmost care and attention.

Chapter 9: Lifestyle Changes for Sustainable Stress and Anxiety Relief

Nutrition and Diet for Balancing Mood

When it comes to managing our mood and emotions, many of us turn to various methods such as essential oils and herbs. However, one aspect that is often overlooked is the role of nutrition and diet in balancing our mood. What we eat can have a profound impact on our overall well-being, including our mental health. In this subchapter, we will explore the connection between nutrition, diet, and mood, and how you can utilize them to enhance your self-care routine with homeopathy.

The Power of Nature: Essential Oils, Herbs, and Homeopathy for Stress and Anxiety Relief

First and foremost, it is important to understand that a healthy diet forms the foundation for emotional well-being. Consuming a well-balanced diet rich in nutrients can help stabilize our moods and reduce symptoms of stress and anxiety. Incorporating whole foods such as fruits, vegetables, whole grains, and lean proteins into our meals provides us with the necessary vitamins and minerals to support a healthy mind.

In particular, certain nutrients have been found to have a direct impact on mood regulation. For example, omega-3 fatty acids found in fatty fish like salmon and walnuts have been shown to reduce symptoms of depression and anxiety. Similarly, foods rich in complex carbohydrates, such as whole grains and legumes, help increase the production of serotonin, the "feel-good" neurotransmitter.

Additionally, incorporating specific herbs and spices into our diet can further enhance our mood-balancing efforts. Turmeric, for instance, contains a compound called curcumin, which has been found to have antidepressant effects. Including turmeric in your cooking or consuming it as a supplement can be beneficial for managing stress and anxiety.

Furthermore, it is important to be mindful of our dietary choices that can negatively impact our mood. Consuming excessive amounts of refined sugars, caffeine, and processed foods can lead to energy crashes and mood swings. Opting for healthier alternatives, such as natural sweeteners like honey or stevia, and replacing caffeinated beverages with herbal teas, can help stabilize your mood throughout the day.

The Power of Nature: Essential Oils, Herbs, and Homeopathy for Stress and Anxiety Relief

In conclusion, nutrition and diet play a vital role in balancing our mood and emotions. By incorporating a well-rounded, nutrient-rich diet with specific mood-enhancing foods, such as omega-3 fatty acids and complex carbohydrates, we can support our mental well-being. Additionally, incorporating herbs and spices like turmeric can further enhance our mood-balancing efforts. By being mindful of our dietary choices and making small changes, we can optimize our self-care routine with homeopathy and experience greater emotional well-being.

Exercise and Physical Activity for Stress Reduction

In the demanding world we live in, stress and anxiety have become unavoidable companions for most individuals. The good news is that there are natural and effective ways to combat these issues, and one of the most powerful tools at our disposal is exercise and physical activity.

Exercise has long been recognized as a potent stress reducer, as it helps release endorphins, the body's natural feel-good chemicals. These endorphins not only boost mood but also act as natural painkillers, promoting a sense of well-being and relaxation. Whether you prefer a vigorous workout or a gentle stroll, any form of physical activity can be beneficial for stress reduction.

Engaging in regular exercise not only helps alleviate the symptoms of stress but also promotes overall mental and physical health. It improves cardiovascular fitness, strengthens the immune system, and increases energy levels, all of which contribute to a more resilient body and mind. Additionally, exercise can enhance cognitive function, memory, and focus, allowing you to better manage stressors and find clarity amidst chaos.

The Power of Nature: Essential Oils, Herbs, and Homeopathy for Stress and Anxiety Relief

When it comes to stress reduction, it's important to find an exercise routine that suits your preferences and lifestyle. Some individuals may enjoy high-intensity activities such as running, kickboxing, or cycling, while others may find solace in more gentle practices like yoga, Pilates, or tai chi. Experimenting with different forms of exercise can help you discover what resonates with you the most and provides the greatest stress-relieving benefits.

To further enhance the stress-reducing effects of exercise, consider incorporating essential oils and herbs into your routine. Essential oils like lavender, chamomile, and bergamot have been shown to have calming properties that can help relax the mind and body. You can diffuse these oils during your workout or apply them topically before or after physical activity for an added sense of tranquility.

Herbs such as ashwagandha, passionflower, and lemon balm are known for their adaptogenic and calming properties. These herbs can be consumed as teas, tinctures, or supplements to support your body's stress response and promote a sense of calmness.

In conclusion, exercise and physical activity are powerful tools for stress reduction. By incorporating regular exercise into your routine and exploring the benefits of essential oils and herbs, you can create a holistic approach to managing stress and anxiety. Remember, self-care is essential, and by prioritizing your well-being, you can navigate life's challenges with resilience and grace.

Adequate Sleep and Rest for Emotional Well-being

The Power of Nature: Essential Oils, Herbs, and Homeopathy for Stress and Anxiety Relief

In the stressful world of today, it is easy to overlook the importance of sleep and rest when it comes to our emotional well-being. However, getting enough sleep and allowing our bodies and minds to rest is crucial for maintaining balance and managing stress and anxiety effectively. In this subchapter, we will explore the role of adequate sleep and rest in promoting emotional well-being and how homeopathy, essential oils, and herbs can support this process.

Sleep is not just a state of unconsciousness; it is a vital process that allows our bodies to repair and rejuvenate. During sleep, our brains consolidate memories, regulate emotions, and process information. When we do not get enough quality sleep, our emotional well-being can suffer. We may find ourselves more irritable, anxious, and prone to stress. Incorporating a regular sleep routine that includes a sufficient number of hours of sleep can significantly improve our emotional resilience.

Homeopathy offers a range of remedies that can address sleep disturbances and promote restful sleep. For example, coffea cruda is a remedy that can help calm an overactive mind, making it easier to fall asleep. Nux vomica is another remedy that can be beneficial for those who have trouble falling asleep due to a racing mind or excessive stress.

In addition to homeopathy, using essential oils and herbs can also support restful sleep. Lavender essential oil is well-known for its relaxing properties and can be diffused in the bedroom or added to a warm bath before bedtime. Chamomile tea is a herbal remedy that has been used for centuries to promote sleep and relaxation. Incorporating these natural remedies into our nighttime routine can create a soothing and calming atmosphere, preparing our bodies and minds for restful sleep.

Remember, sleep and rest are not signs of laziness but essential components of self-care. By prioritizing adequate sleep and rest, we can better manage stress and anxiety, leading to improved emotional well-being. Through the use of homeopathy, essential oils, and herbs, we have powerful tools at our disposal to enhance our sleep and rest experience. By incorporating these practices into our self-care routine, we can reap the benefits of a well-rested mind and body, ultimately leading to a happier and healthier life.

Managing Time and Prioritizing Self-Care

With the fast pace of our everyday lives, it can be challenging to find time for self-care. However, taking care of ourselves is crucial for our overall well-being, especially when dealing with stress and anxiety. This subchapter aims to provide individuals interested in self-care with homeopathy practical strategies for managing time effectively and incorporating essential oils and herbs into their daily routines for stress and anxiety relief.

One of the first steps towards managing time is to identify our priorities. By understanding what matters most to us, we can allocate our time and energy accordingly. It is essential to set realistic goals and establish a clear schedule that allows for self-care activities. This includes allocating specific time slots for using essential oils and herbs, such as creating a calming aromatherapy routine or consuming herbal teas known for their stress-relieving properties.

Another effective strategy for managing time is to eliminate or delegate non-essential tasks. By learning to say no and setting boundaries, we can free up time for self-care activities. It is crucial to remember that self-care is not selfish; it is an investment in our overall well-being. Utilizing essential oils and herbs can be an excellent way to take care of ourselves, as they have been used for centuries to promote relaxation and alleviate stress and anxiety.

Essential oils, such as lavender, chamomile, and bergamot, have calming properties that can help reduce anxiety and promote better sleep. Incorporating these oils into our daily routine, whether through diffusing them in the air or adding a few drops to a bath, can provide a much-needed sense of relaxation and rejuvenation.

Similarly, herbs like valerian root, passionflower, and lemon balm have been used traditionally to reduce stress and anxiety. Creating herbal infusions or tinctures and incorporating them into our daily routine can help us combat the negative effects of stress and promote a greater sense of calm and well-being.

In conclusion, managing time effectively and prioritizing self-care is crucial for individuals interested in utilizing homeopathy for stress and anxiety relief. By identifying priorities, setting boundaries, and incorporating essential oils and herbs into our daily routines, we can create a healthier and more balanced lifestyle. Remember, self-care is not a luxury but a necessity, and by investing in ourselves, we can better navigate the challenges of modern life and achieve a greater sense of well-being.

Cultivating Healthy Relationships and Boundaries

The Power of Nature: Essential Oils, Herbs, and Homeopathy for Stress and Anxiety Relief

In our quest for stress and anxiety relief, it is essential that we not overlook the impact of our relationships and the boundaries we set within them. The power of nature, including essential oils, herbs, and homeopathy, extends beyond physical well-being; it can also contribute to cultivating healthier relationships and establishing boundaries that promote personal growth and emotional balance.

Relationships are the cornerstone of our lives, and they can greatly influence our stress levels and overall well-being. By harnessing the power of essential oils and herbs, we can enhance our emotional resilience, improve communication, and foster deeper connections with our loved ones. For instance, lavender essential oil is renowned for its calming properties, making it an excellent tool for diffusing tension during conflicts or heated discussions. Similarly, herbs like chamomile and passionflower can help reduce anxiety and promote relaxation, creating a more serene environment for open and honest communication.

However, cultivating healthy relationships isn't just about using essential oils and herbs as quick fixes. It requires a holistic approach that involves setting and respecting boundaries. Establishing boundaries is crucial for maintaining emotional well-being and preventing stress and anxiety from seeping into our relationships. Homeopathy can provide valuable support in this regard. Remedies like Ignatia and Natrum Muriaticum can help individuals address emotional wounds, heal from past traumas, and gain the strength to set healthy boundaries with others.

Additionally, the practice of self-care with homeopathy encourages individuals to prioritize their own needs and well-being. By taking the time to care for ourselves, we can foster a sense of self-worth and establish clear boundaries that protect our mental and emotional health. Essential oils and herbs can be incorporated into self-care routines to further promote relaxation and release stress. For example, a warm bath infused with lavender essential oil can provide a soothing escape from the demands of everyday life, allowing us to recharge and be more present in our relationships.

In conclusion, integrating essential oils, herbs, and homeopathy into our self-care practices can significantly contribute to cultivating healthy relationships and boundaries. By utilizing the power of nature, we can enhance emotional resilience, improve communication, and protect our mental and emotional well-being. Remember, self-care is not selfish; it is a necessary foundation for nurturing meaningful connections and finding balance in our lives.

Chapter 10: Integrating Natural Remedies into Everyday Life

Incorporating Essential Oils into Household Products

If you're someone who is interested in self-care with homeopathy, you'll be delighted to learn about the incredible benefits of incorporating essential oils into your household products. Essential oils have been used for centuries for their therapeutic properties, and they can be a powerful tool in relieving stress and anxiety in your daily life.

The Power of Nature: Essential Oils, Herbs, and Homeopathy for Stress and Anxiety Relief

When it comes to utilizing essential oils and herbs for stress and anxiety relief, it's important to understand that the power of nature lies in their natural properties. These oils are derived from plants and contain concentrated extracts that have been proven to have a positive impact on our mental and emotional well-being.

One effective way to incorporate essential oils into your household products is by making your own cleaning solutions. Commercial cleaning products often contain harsh chemicals that can be irritating to your senses, exacerbating stress and anxiety. By creating your own cleaning products using essential oils, you not only eliminate exposure to toxins but also benefit from the calming and soothing effects of these oils.

For example, you can add a few drops of lavender essential oil to your homemade laundry detergent. Lavender is well-known for its relaxing properties and can help promote a sense of tranquility while doing your laundry. Similarly, you can infuse your all-purpose cleaner with lemon essential oil, which is not only a powerful disinfectant but also has uplifting properties that can help combat stress.

Another way to incorporate essential oils into your household products is by creating natural air fresheners. Many commercial air fresheners contain synthetic fragrances that can be overwhelming and even trigger anxiety in some individuals. By using essential oils such as peppermint or eucalyptus, you can create a refreshing and invigorating atmosphere in your home, promoting a sense of calmness and balance.

In addition to cleaning solutions and air fresheners, essential oils can also be added to bath and body products. A relaxing bath infused with lavender or chamomile essential oil can be a wonderful way to unwind after a long day and release built-up tension. You can also create your own massage oils using essential oils known for their stress-relieving properties, such as bergamot or ylang-ylang.

Incorporating essential oils into your household products is not only a natural and effective way to combat stress and anxiety but also allows you to customize your self-care routine to suit your individual needs. By harnessing the power of nature, you can create a harmonious environment that promotes relaxation, balance, and overall well-being.

Creating Herbal Remedies for Daily Wellness

In our current stressful modern world, finding ways to support our daily wellness is essential. Many individuals are turning to natural remedies like essential oils and herbs to help manage stress and anxiety. In this subchapter, we will explore the power of nature and learn how to create herbal remedies that promote overall well-being.

Herbs have been used for centuries to support the body's natural healing abilities. By harnessing the therapeutic properties of various plants, we can create personalized remedies that address our unique needs. When it comes to stress and anxiety relief, there are several herbs that have proven to be effective.

One such herb is lavender. Known for its calming and relaxing properties, lavender can help reduce stress and promote a restful sleep. By infusing dried lavender flowers in carrier oils such as jojoba or almond oil, we can create a soothing massage oil or a calming bath soak.

Another powerful herb for daily wellness is chamomile. This gentle herb has been used for centuries to ease tension and promote relaxation. By brewing chamomile tea and adding a few drops of lemon balm essential oil, we can create a comforting blend that can be enjoyed throughout the day.

In addition to herbs, essential oils can also play a significant role in managing stress and anxiety. Oils like bergamot, ylang-ylang, and frankincense have been shown to have uplifting and calming effects on the mind and body. By blending these oils with a carrier oil, we can create a personal aromatherapy rollerball that can be applied to pulse points whenever needed.

When creating herbal remedies for daily wellness, it is crucial to remember that everyone's needs are unique. Experimentation and personalization are key in finding the right combination of herbs and essential oils that work best for you. Start by researching different herbs and their properties, and consult with a qualified herbalist or aromatherapist for guidance.

By incorporating herbal remedies into our daily routines, we can proactively support our mental and emotional well-being. Nature provides us with a vast array of tools to manage stress and anxiety, and by harnessing their power, we can find a sense of balance and tranquility in our lives.

Building a Homeopathic First Aid Kit

For individuals interested in self-care with homeopathy, having a reliable first aid kit is essential. In this subchapter, we will guide you through the process of building a homeopathic first aid kit that can help alleviate stress and anxiety. By understanding how to utilize essential oils and herbs in various situations, you can effectively manage your well-being and promote a sense of calm in your daily life.

The Power of Nature: Essential Oils, Herbs, and Homeopathy for Stress and Anxiety Relief

When it comes to addressing stress and anxiety, essential oils play a vital role. Lavender oil, for instance, is known for its calming properties and can be used to reduce nervousness and promote relaxation. Similarly, bergamot oil can uplift your mood and relieve anxiety. Including these essential oils in your first aid kit can provide you with natural remedies to combat stress-inducing situations.

Herbs can also be powerful allies in managing stress and anxiety. One such herb is chamomile, which has been used for centuries to soothe nerves and promote sleep. St. John's Wort is another herbal remedy known for its ability to alleviate mild to moderate depression and anxiety. By incorporating these herbs into your first aid kit, you can have quick and convenient access to nature's stress-relieving wonders.

In addition to essential oils and herbs, homeopathy offers a range of remedies that can effectively address stress and anxiety. Ignatia, for example, is often used for emotional distress, including grief and anxiety. Aconite is useful for sudden panic attacks and restlessness, while Gelsemium is beneficial for anticipatory anxiety and stage fright. By including these homeopathic remedies in your first aid kit, you can have a well-rounded approach to managing stress and anxiety.

When assembling your homeopathic first aid kit, consider including essential oils such as lavender and bergamot, as well as herbs like chamomile and St. John's Wort. Additionally, stock up on homeopathic remedies like Ignatia, Aconite, and Gelsemium. With these natural tools at your disposal, you can take control of your well-being and find relief from stress and anxiety whenever they arise.

Remember, self-care is a journey, and building a homeopathic first aid kit is just one step towards achieving a balanced and peaceful lifestyle. By exploring the power of nature through essential oils, herbs, and homeopathy, you can unlock the potential for stress and anxiety relief, allowing you to live your life to the fullest.

Sharing the Benefits of Natural Remedies with Family and Friends

In the realm of self-care with homeopathy, one of the most rewarding aspects is being able to share the incredible benefits of natural remedies with our loved ones. Whether it's our family, friends, or even acquaintances, spreading the knowledge and promoting the use of essential oils, herbs, and homeopathy for stress and anxiety relief can be a game-changer in their lives.

When we discover the power of nature's remedies, it becomes our responsibility to educate others and help them tap into the vast potential of these healing modalities. Here are some ways you can effectively share the benefits of natural remedies with your loved ones:

1. Start with Personal Experience: Begin by sharing your own journey towards stress and anxiety relief through essential oils, herbs, and homeopathy. Describe the positive impact these natural remedies have had on your well-being, emphasizing the non-invasive and holistic approach they offer.

2. Education and Awareness: Offer to educate your family and friends about the different essential oils, herbs, and homeopathic remedies that specifically target stress and anxiety. Explain how they work, their safety profiles, and any precautions to be aware of. Provide them with credible resources and references to deepen their understanding.

3. DIY Workshops: Organize small workshops or gatherings where you can teach your loved ones how to create their own stress-relieving blends or herbal remedies. This hands-on approach allows them to experience the process firsthand and empowers them to take control of their own well-being.

4. Gift the Power of Nature: Consider giving essential oil diffusers, starter kits, or herbal wellness baskets as gifts to your family and friends. This not only introduces them to the world of natural remedies but also encourages them to incorporate self-care into their daily lives.

5. Share Success Stories: Collect testimonials from individuals who have benefited from using essential oils, herbs, and homeopathy for stress and anxiety relief. These success stories can be incredibly inspiring and serve as proof of the efficacy of natural remedies.

Remember, sharing the benefits of natural remedies should be done with respect and without imposing one's beliefs on others. Each person has their own journey, and it's important to approach them with empathy and understanding. By imparting knowledge and encouraging exploration, you are giving your loved ones the tools they need to embark on their own path towards stress and anxiety relief.

In conclusion, sharing the benefits of natural remedies with family and friends is a beautiful way to spread the power of nature's healing abilities. By educating, inspiring, and providing practical tools, you can help others discover the transformative potential of essential oils, herbs, and homeopathy in their own self-care journeys. Together, we can create a community that embraces and utilizes the incredible gifts nature has to offer.

Embracing Nature's Healing Power for Long-Term Well-being

In our stressful modern lives, finding effective ways to manage stress and anxiety has become increasingly crucial. While pharmaceutical solutions are readily available, many individuals are now seeking natural alternatives for self-care and long-term well-being. This subchapter aims to explore the power of nature in relieving stress and anxiety through the utilization of essential oils, herbs, and homeopathy.

Nature has always been a source of healing and rejuvenation. Essential oils, extracted from various plants, possess potent therapeutic properties that can positively impact our mental and emotional well-being. Lavender, for instance, is known for its calming and relaxing effects. By diffusing lavender essential oil or adding a few drops to a warm bath, individuals can create a serene and tranquil environment to alleviate stress and anxiety.

In addition to essential oils, herbs have been used for centuries to promote well-being and restore balance. Adaptogenic herbs such as ashwagandha and holy basil help the body adapt to stress and improve resilience. These herbs can be consumed in the form of teas, tinctures, or supplements to support the body's natural stress response system.

Homeopathy, a system of alternative medicine, utilizes highly diluted substances to stimulate the body's natural healing process. Remedies such as Ignatia and Gelsemium are commonly used for anxiety relief. Homeopathy treats the individual as a whole, considering their unique symptoms and emotional state, making it a personalized and effective approach to managing stress and anxiety.

By embracing nature's healing power, individuals can achieve long-term well-being and reduce reliance on pharmaceutical interventions. Incorporating essential oils, herbs, and homeopathy into a self-care routine can provide a holistic approach to stress and anxiety relief. However, it is important to note that the effectiveness of these natural remedies may vary from person to person, and consulting with a qualified healthcare practitioner is recommended.

To fully utilize essential oils and herbs for stress and anxiety relief, it is essential to understand their properties, correct usage, and potential interactions. This subchapter will provide comprehensive information, including practical tips, recipes, and precautions, to ensure individuals can safely and effectively incorporate these natural remedies into their self-care routine.

In conclusion, this subchapter highlights the immense potential of nature in promoting long-term well-being and relieving stress and anxiety. By embracing essential oils, herbs, and homeopathy, individuals interested in self-care with homeopathy can discover natural and holistic approaches to enhance their mental and emotional health. Through the power of nature, we can find balance, harmony, and a renewed sense of calm in our lives.

Conclusion: Embracing Self-Care with Natural Remedies for Stress and Anxiety Relief

In this journey of exploring the power of nature and its ability to provide relief from stress and anxiety, we have delved into the world of essential oils, herbs, and homeopathy. Throughout this book, we have discovered the incredible potential of these natural remedies in promoting emotional well-being and restoring balance in our lives.

The Power of Nature: Essential Oils, Herbs, and Homeopathy for Stress and Anxiety Relief

For individuals interested in self-care with homeopathy, this subchapter serves as a culmination of all the knowledge and insights we have gained so far. It is a reminder of the transformative potential that lies within these natural remedies and how they can be utilized to alleviate stress and anxiety.

One of the most significant takeaways from this book is the importance of embracing self-care as an integral part of our lives. Stress and anxiety are pervasive in today's fast-paced world, and it is crucial to prioritize our mental and emotional well-being. By incorporating natural remedies into our self-care routines, we can create a sanctuary of peace and tranquility amidst the chaos.

Essential oils have proven to be powerful allies in reducing stress and anxiety. Whether it is the soothing aroma of lavender, the uplifting scent of citrus, or the grounding properties of frankincense, these oils have the ability to calm our minds and promote relaxation. By creating personalized blends and incorporating them into our daily rituals, we can harness the therapeutic benefits of essential oils and find solace in their gentle embrace.

Herbs, too, have played a significant role in our journey towards stress and anxiety relief. From chamomile and passionflower to valerian and lemon balm, these herbal allies have been used for centuries to calm the mind, ease tension, and promote restful sleep. Whether consumed as teas, tinctures, or in other forms, herbs offer a holistic approach to combating stress and anxiety, gently soothing our frayed nerves and restoring harmony within.

The Power of Nature: Essential Oils, Herbs, and Homeopathy for Stress and Anxiety Relief

Lastly, we explored the principles of homeopathy, a powerful system of medicine that recognizes the body's innate ability to heal itself. By using highly diluted substances derived from nature, homeopathy aims to stimulate the body's vital force and restore balance on a deep level. Whether it is Ignatia for grief, Arsenicum album for restlessness, or Aconitum napellus for acute anxiety, homeopathy offers individualized remedies that can address the underlying causes of stress and anxiety.

In conclusion, the power of nature is vast and awe-inspiring. By embracing self-care with natural remedies such as essential oils, herbs, and homeopathy, we can embark on a transformative journey towards stress and anxiety relief. Let us remember to prioritize our well-being and create space for healing, allowing the magic of nature to guide us towards inner peace and emotional harmony.